PARADISE OF OLIVE OIL

Natural and Easy tips with Olive oil to regain your

beauty charms of your Hair, Skin and Nails

I0440519

AVA COLLINS

TABLE OF CONTENTS

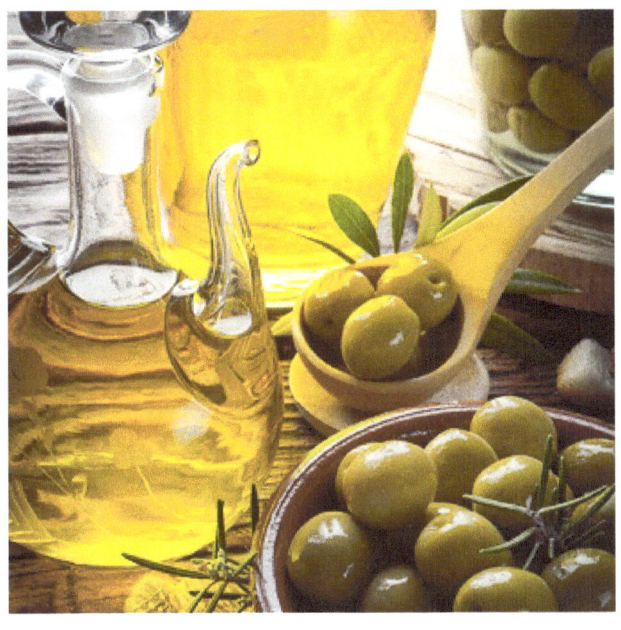

Many of the latest "miracle in a jar" options are marketed as high-end, but costly, solutions to everyday challenges: how to keep skin moisturized, hair healthy, and facial skin free of wrinkles. Some of the most popular products, promoted as "natural" solutions, even incorporate olive oil as a key ingredient in their formulas.

But what many don't realize is something that people living millennia ago in ancient times took for granted; that olive oil, all by itself, is one of the best beauty secrets. In addition to being a natural, hypoallergenic way to moisturize skin, hair and nails. Olive oil has the added advantage of providing strong antioxidants, like Vitamins A and E that help repair and renew skin roots that has been damaged from overexposure to sun, air pollution, and other modern-day environmental hazards – like cigarette smoke and fast food. These antioxidants have the natural ability to stimulate cells and return skin and hair to a firmer, smoother, and healthier state.

To provide a slightly more scientific explanation, this damage is related to the destructive activity of oxygen-related free radicals produced by skin cells. Polyphenolic components of olive oil have been compared to traditional antioxidants, such as tocopherols, used by the pharmaceutical and cosmetic industry to prevent skin and hair damage. There are a number of simple and inexpensive ways to get the best skin care and beauty benefits out of a single bottle of olive oil. The rich emollients in olive oil allow just a little to go a long way.

OLIVE OIL TREATMNET FOR HAIR

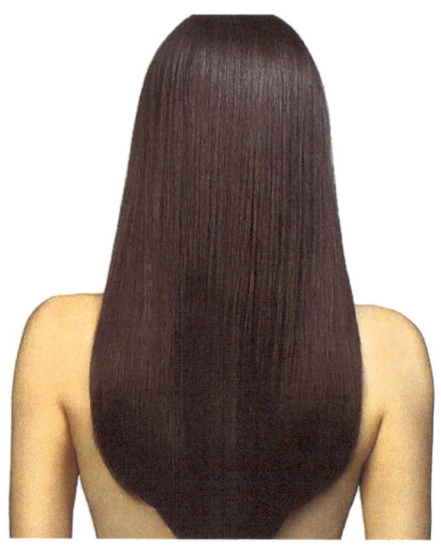

There are many people out there who dream of having the same beautiful hair that they see on television and in magazines. And many of these people are willing to try just about anything that promises beautiful, glowing hair. This makes many people ask, is olive oil good for hair? When you use olive oil for a hair conditioner, you will see a difference in your hair. Your hair is going to be more vibrant, stronger and healthier looking overall.

Olive oil is known to be one of the best natural remedies for promoting the growth of good hair and skin and overall body *health. This is because olive oil is rich in polyphenols which have anti bacterial and anti fungal properties.*

Hence, some of the most effective home remedies for hair involve the use of olive oil as it leaves the hair looking healthier and more manageable.

When using olive oil on your hair, the oil coats each strand, making it stronger and shinier. With these benefits it is easy to see that the use of olive oil on hair is a great decision.

Olive oil hair treatment not only benefits the hair but also results in the scalp becoming cleaner. Olive oil hair conditioning is apt for curly or very dry hair as it tends to smoothen out frizzy and dry hair but does not leave any build up which is found in other hair conditioning treatments. Hence, plenty of people even use olive oil as a serum to tame frizzy hair.

HAIR FALL REMEDIES FROM OLIVE OIL:

Is olive oil good for hair, Yes, just as olive oil acts as an effective moisturizing agent on your skin, it has similar benefits on the hair too. Olive oil works wonders for dry damaged hair that can otherwise cause other hair problems, such as split ends and frizzy hair. To nurture those dry manes give your hair a hot olive oil hair massage. Make it sure that olive oil is not heated too much and too long, as it will lose its benefits.

- One of the common olive oil hair remedies for hair re-growth involves mixing one beaten egg in 3/4 cup of olive oil and then applying this mixture to the hair after it is shampooed and is still wet. This mixture should be allowed to remain on the hair for at least 45 minutes before washing it off with a mild shampoo.

  Thus not only is olive oil good for hair growth but it is also used as an excellent conditioner that also aids in increasing hair volume.

- **Olive Oil Hair Treatment – Eggs And Olive Oil For Hair:** This olive oil hair mask / treatment is fast and easy to prepare and takes only 15 minutes to apply and through with it. Blend 1 egg yolk with 2 tablespoons of olive oil and a teaspoon of lemon juice. Massage your hair and keep it there for about 15 minutes. Shampoo and condition your hair as usual. Your hair will look and feel shinier and soft.

  Olive oil has vitamin E and A, as well as antioxidants that can help to make the hair strands stronger and shinier. Studies have shown that regular use of olive oil as a conditioner can add needed nutrition back into each strand of hair and help with the shine. Olive oil for hair growth is also an added positive when using regularly.

- **All Alone Olive Oil Hair Treatment:** This olive oil hair mask / treatment is the most easy to follow. Simply massage slightly warmed up olive oil on your hair. Allow it to sit on your tresses for about an hour, then shampoo and condition as you normally do. If after shampoo your hair still feels oily, you may need to do shampoo twice to get rid of greasiness.

Your hair will look and feel healthier and shiny after this olive oil hair treatment.

- Those who have dry, frizzy or split ends can massage their tresses with lightly warmed olive oil. As said earlier, don't heat the olive oil too much, as it loses its properties even at low temperature.

- **Prevent Bacterial and Fungal Infections:** Clogging of pores on scalp can have minor to major problems when they get contaminated with bacteria or fungi. These bacteria and fungi provides nourishment and gives suitable environment for hair lice growth and dandruff. And can be the major cause of hair loss or hair fall. If the scalp is getting tender and there are some red spots you must visit a dermatologist. Along with the scalp, hair can get red. Although, bacteria is present all the time but the one mentioned is scalp-friendly. Irritation on scalp and redness can be the result of some harmful bacteria
replacing normal one. Regularly oiling hair with honey gives you anti-bacterial treatment and provides scalp the necessary elements to stay healthy and well hydrated.

- **Olive Oil Hair Treatment – Eggs And Olive Oil For Hair:** This olive oil hair mask / treatment is fast and easy to prepare and takes only 15 minutes to apply and through with it. Blend 1 egg yolk with 2 tablespoons of olive oil and a teaspoon of lemon juice. Massage your hair and keep it there for about 15 minutes. Shampoo and condition your hair as usual. Your hair will look and feel shinier and soft.

  Olive oil has vitamin E and A, as well as antioxidants that can help to make the hair strands stronger and shinier. Studies have shown that regular use of olive oil as a conditioner can add needed nutrition back into each strand of hair and help with the shine. Olive oil for hair growth is also an added positive when using regularly.

- **All Alone Olive Oil Hair Treatment:** This olive oil hair mask / treatment is the most easy to follow. Simply massage slightly warmed up olive oil on your hair. Allow it to sit on your tresses for about an hour, then shampoo and condition as you normally do. If after shampoo your hair still feels oily, you may need to do shampoo twice to get rid of greasiness.

Your hair will look and feel healthier and shiny after this olive oil hair treatment.

- Those who have dry, frizzy or split ends can massage their tresses with lightly warmed olive oil. As said earlier, don't heat the olive oil too much, as it loses its properties even at low temperature.

- **Prevent Bacterial and Fungal Infections:** Clogging of pores on scalp can have minor to major problems when they get contaminated with bacteria or fungi. These bacteria and fungi provides nourishment and gives suitable environment for hair lice growth and dandruff. And can be the major cause of hair loss or hair fall. If the scalp is getting tender and there are some red spots you must visit a dermatologist. Along with the scalp, hair can get red. Although, bacteria is present all the time but the one mentioned is scalp-friendly. Irritation on scalp and redness can be the result of some harmful bacteria replacing normal one. Regularly oiling hair with honey gives you anti-bacterial treatment and provides scalp the necessary elements to stay healthy and well hydrated.

- **Olive Oil For Lice Treatment:** A lesser known fact about olive oil is that it is also effective in tackling the problem of hair lice without the agony and irritation associated with other commercial hair lice removal products. Additionally, olive oil also improves the elasticity of hair and prevents hair breakage.

- **Decrease in Dandruff:** Dandruff often results due to a dry scalp, which then becomes irritated and leads to other concerns. With the use of olive oil, you can moisturize the scalp, which aids in decreasing dandruff.

  Olive oil is also known to have emollient properties thereby minimizing hair loss and factors causing hair loss such as dandruff. Olive oil hair re-growth treatment involves the regular use of olive oil directly on the hair and on the scalp as it helps solves the problem of brittle hair and also regularly massaging the scalp with olive oil tends to stimulate the scalp and promote hair growth.

- **Split Ends:** When the weather is dry and cold, many people experience dry and frizzy hair, especially on the ends of each strand. When this occurs, the hair looks messy, in spite of the fact that the hairstyle may be new. Olive oil can help subdue the hair that is reacting to this dry and cold weather by adding the extra moisture that the hair needs.

- **Prevents Greying and acts as a protective sheath:** Premature-greying of hair is common in youngsters and adults. It occurs due to lack of vitamins and protein in the food digested. However, there may be reasons genetically that leads to graying of hair. Melanin present in the skin gives hair its color, as it does to skin. Melanin is a skin pigment that decides color of hair. High amount of melanin present in scalp gives dark color to hair while its lack causes graying. It is the deficiency of Vitamin B 12 that results in graying. Regularly oiling and massaging thus helps to retain the color of your hair, and thus giving you black and shining hair. Also, hair are prevented from harmful rays of sunlight by forming a protective sheath around the hair protein. UV rays are blocked by the oil that nourishes hair. Nourished hair are more resistant to harmful rays.

Methods of using Olive Oil:

Applying olive oil to your hair will mean following a few steps in order to use it properly to get the best benefits for your hair:

1. Place the olive oil into a microwaveable bowl or cup to warm up. A half cup is often the recommended amount to use. Warm this up to the point that it is warm, but not too hot.

2. While warm, put one tablespoon of the olive oil onto the palms of your hands and rub together.

3. Starting at the roots of your hair, massage the oil into the scalp with your hands. Continue this process until you get to the tips of the hair, putting more olive oil on the hands when this is needed.

4. Once all the hair has been saturated, wrap your hair with a shower cap or use an old towel to wrap your head and hold the heat in the olive oil.

5. Let the olive stay on the hair for 5 minutes for a light conditioning, or 45 minutes for a deeper conditioning.

6. Rinse the oil from the hair, then shampoo and condition as you normally would.

Although there are a number of other benefits of regularly oiling and massaging, it provide basic nourishment for hair growth. Oil act as lubricant on hair preventing it from harsh environment. Hair oil is a necessary for volume and strength, it is thus called the grandma's treatment.

Oil you hair regularly with lure oils to see the change yourself.....

OLIVE OIL TREATMNET FOR SKIN

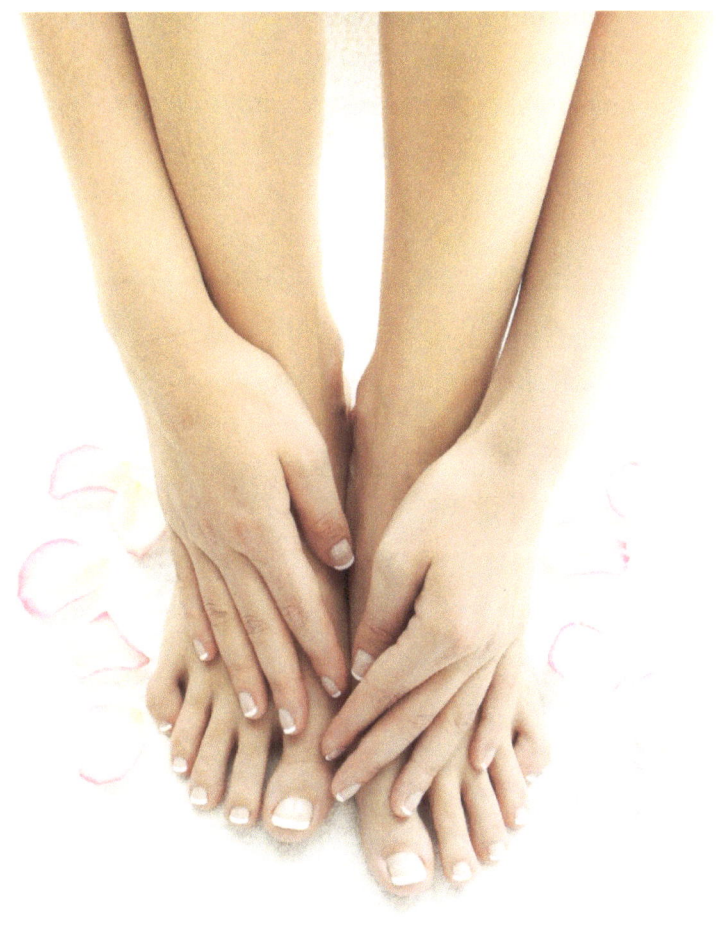

One of the favorite natural beauty products of the beauty queen Cleopatra was the Extra Virgin Olive Oil (hereinafter referred to as Olive Oil). Over the

last decade, many beauticians are advocating the use of olive oil due to its many beauty benefits, but the fact is that this natural ingredient has been used on the body since centuries. It was commonly used in Egypt as a cosmetic, is still going strong and is being used in cosmetic industry even now.

Oil cleansing is the process of using oil (instead of soap or a cleanser) to dissolve and remove dirt on the skin.

Is Olive Oil Good For Skin? The answer is a big yes!! Olive oil's chemical structure is more close to the skin's natural oil as compared to that of any other natural oil, making olive oil good for skin.

Methods of Using Olive Oil:

1. Olive Oil Bath: Do you know beauty secret of Sophia Loren, the Italian gorgeous actress – she loved taking olive oil bath.

OLIVE OIL TREATMNET FOR SKIN

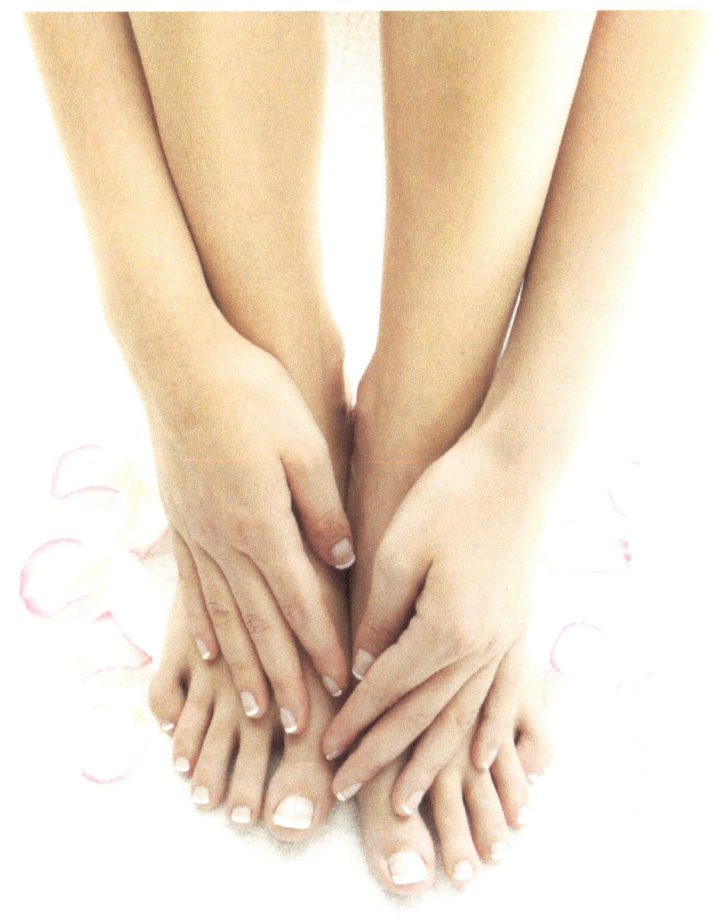

One of the favorite natural beauty products of the

beauty queen Cleopatra was the Extra Virgin Olive

Oil (hereinafter referred to as Olive Oil). Over the

last decade, many beauticians are advocating the use of olive oil due to its many beauty benefits, but the fact is that this natural ingredient has been used on the body since centuries. It was commonly used in Egypt as a cosmetic, is still going strong and is being used in cosmetic industry even now.

Oil cleansing is the process of using oil (instead of soap or a cleanser) to dissolve and remove dirt on the skin.

Is Olive Oil Good For Skin? The answer is a big yes!! Olive oil's chemical structure is more close to the skin's natural oil as compared to that of any other natural oil, making olive oil good for skin.

Methods of Using Olive Oil:

1. Olive Oil Bath: Do you know beauty secret of Sophia Loren, the Italian gorgeous actress – she loved taking olive oil bath.

- The simplest way to prepare olive oil bath is just to add 5 tablespoons of extra virgin olive oil into your bathtub and it's done! If you like, you may add more. This is a simple beauty trick to make your skin soft and smooth.

- Another simple way to have olive oil on skin is that you just massage your body with extra virgin oil before taking bath. After you are through with your bath, pat dry your skin and wipe away the excess oil. Wow!! You will feel your skin as incredibly soft and smooth, just like a baby-skin.

2. Olive Oil Body Lotion: Try olive oil as a body lotion. It's all natural and wonderfully very effective. Apply it all over your body, while in the shower, right after you use the shower gel. You will feel your skin amazingly soft and smooth. This is another simple way to make your skin look perfect, healthy and tender to touch.

3. Olive Oil – A Natural Makeup Remover: It serves dual purpose. While gently removing makeup, it nourishes your skin as well. Just put a dab of olive oil on a cotton ball or pad, and gently wipe out all the makeup from your face. If you want to remove heavy makeup, first massage gently olive oil all over your face, and then wipe away all the makeup with a soft washcloth soaked with warm water. If needed, repeat it a couple of times and make it sure to do it gently – never rub your skin harshly. Rinse your face with warm water followed by a splash with cold water. Cold water will not only close your skin pores, but stimulate the blood circulation as well.

4. Olive Oil For Sensitive Skin: It is a very good option for those even having sensitive skin. If you are concerned about the oiliness it leaves behind, that hitch can simply be resolved by washing your face with a face wash of your choice after you have removed makeup with olive oil. This will also make sure that there are no traces of makeup left behind on your face.

Tip: You can use olive oil as a gentle eye makeup remover too. It is so effective that even you can remove waterproof makeup with its help.

5. Olive Oil Rejuvenates Skin: The prime reason behind beauty benefits of olive oil is that it is packed with healthy fats and phenolic antioxidant vitamin E accompanied by squalene and oleic acids.

They work to get rid of free radicals and repair the damage done because of any skin's exposure to the sun.

6. Olive Oil As Stretch Marks Home Remedy: Olive oil helps in regeneration of skin and increasing elasticity of the skin as well. Massage olive oil over the affected areas at least three times a week to improve the elasticity of the skin and its regenerative abilities, which will help heal the affected skin. This will not only prevent formation of new stretch marks, but will also work to reduce and lighten the existing ones slightly.

7. Olive Oil To Prevent Premature Ageing: Olive oil contains hydroxytyrosol and vitamin E that act on the skin to prevent skin cells degeneration, thus olive oil helps in preventing premature ageing. Further, olive oil also has squalene acid that works to increase the elasticity of the skin, thus preventing sagging of the skin and making it firm, young and healthy.

8. Olive Oil As Sunscreen: Mix equal amounts of olive oil and tea decoction (tea boiled in water and strained). Apply this mixture all over your body and face. Let it sit there for about an hour, and then rinse it off (don't wash), so as to leave a residue on your skin. This will work as a natural sunscreen.

Art of Olive oil-cleansing:

The skin of my adult years has been pretty problem-free. It's neither too dry nor too oily, and I've been pretty content with my 15-year hiatus of using Cataphyll or its generic equivalent. But since I turned 30 a few years ago, I've noticed that my skin has become... blah. Kinda dull. Losing its vibrancy. A little cloudy. It's also been dry and tight after washing, and even moisturizing wasn't helping much.

Like your hair, the sebum that the skin secretes is actually good for your skin — it's there to protect it from the outside environment, and to keep harmful things from seeping in. Since water doesn't break up oil, most commercial cleansers are marketed with the "oil free" stamp of approval, making them easy to splash off.

When skin's natural oils are removed, the body's reaction is to compensate by producing more oil, much like shampoo does with our hair. Or if your skin is dry, it's because all the oil has been stripped away, and your body doesn't compensate by replenishing it (that was my case).

"**Oil dissolves oil.** One of the most basic principles of chemistry is that "like dissolves like." The best way to dissolve a non-polar solvent like sebum/oil, is by using another non-polar solvent similar in composition: other oils. By using the right oils, you can cleanse your pores of dirt and bacteria naturally, gently and effectively, while replacing the dirty oil with beneficial ones extracted from natural botanicals, vegetables and fruit that **heal, protect and nourish your skin**. When done properly and consistently, the OCM can clear the skin from issues like oily skin, dry skin, sensitive skin, blackheads, whiteheads and other problems caused by mild to moderate acne–while leaving your skin healthy, balanced and properly moisturized."

So in essence, good-quality oil is the perfect substance for cleaning sensitive skin, such as on our face, because **it helps gently remove the dirty oil and replaces it with good, nourishing, healing oil**.

Natural Beauty Benefits Of Olive Oil For Skin:

- It works as an effective natural moisturizer, even on the dry skin.

- You can use olive oil to moisturize even the super dry skin prone areas, such as elbows and knees.

- Olive oil can regenerate skin tissues and therefore you can use it regularly to keep your skin young, firm and free from wrinkles and fine lines.

- You can make a homemade moisturizer by mixing well together equal parts of oil and water in a jar. Massage your skin with this solution and rinse it off with lukewarm water.

- Try this olive oil moisturizing mask. Blend together 1 tablespoon of honey, 1 tablespoon of olive oil and yolk of one egg. Apply on a clean face, leaving it there for 15-20 minutes. Rinse it off with lukewarm water. This will not only moisturize your skin, but will maintain your natural skin tone too.

- Try this olive oil mask to rejuvenate your skin. Make a paste of olive oil and mashed ripe avocados. Apply this mask on to your face for 20-25 minutes, and then rinse it off.

- If you have super dry skin, apply olive oil as a night cream. Apply a small amount of olive oil on your face and let it sit there for overnight. Wake up in the morning with soft and smooth skin.

- Effective blood circulation is necessary for having natural glow on your skin. Massage olive oil on your body to augment the blood circulation to keep your skin moisturized and young.

Olive Oil For Your Body:

- **Ear Wax Remedy:** A great mom's remedy! If you have wax buildup, you can drizzle olive oil into your ear to help flush it out. For three nights, put a few drops into your ears to help clean them out.

- **Shaving Cream:** A hydrating pre-shave ritual: apply olive oil directly to legs, let it absorb a bit (or your razor will clog), then shave. You avoid razor burn, bumps and irritation.

- **Antibacterial Ointment:** Especially good for burns, take olive oil and mix in lavender, soothing calendula, and antiseptic tea tree oil to moisturize, protect and prevent scarring.

- **Sunburn Salve:** Take equal parts olive oil and white vinegar and pour into a warm bath to help soothe and heal sun burn skin. After the bath, apply olive oil directly to the skin to hydrate and prevent peeling.

- **Eczema and Itchy Skin Remedy:** Apply olive oil directly to affected areas. You can spruce up the formula by adding chamomile essential oil, a known anti-itching and irritation agent. Bonus: the oil helps calm redness.

- **Bath Oil:** Pour olive oil directly in the bath for an incredibly moisturizing treatment. If that's too slippery for you, massage the oil directly into the skin and then get into a warm bath with all your usual bath-time elements.

- **Hand and Foot Care:** Apply olive oil to everything from ragged cuticles (soak your fingers in a bowl of olive oil and water) to cracked heel (apply olive oil directly and then put on some socks to help seal it in!), olive oil is a miracle worker. You can even use a mixture of extra virgin olive oil (EVOO) and lemon juice to remove nail polish stains.

- **Massage Oil:** Take EVOO, coconut oil, and mix in a smaller amount of jojoba, almond oil or vitamin E oil to help keep your skin (or a client's) smooth and soft.

- **Stretch Marks Salve:** Who knew applying olive oil topically could help get rid of stretch marks? It helps regenerate skin as well as moisturize so those tiny tears don't add up. Apply generously every morning to affected areas.

OLIVE OIL FOR NAILS

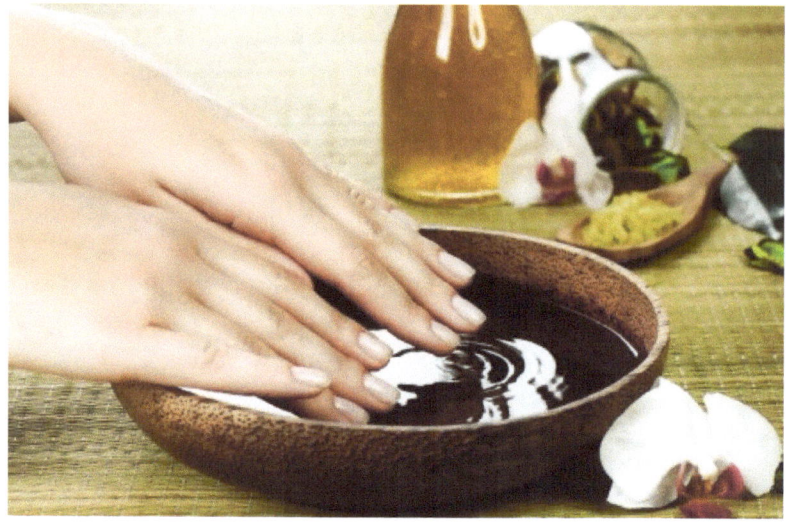

Used globally for its unique flavor and taste, olive oil is appreciated for its myriad health benefits besides a few other interestingly surprising uses at home as well as on the body. Let us check how you can use olive oil to get and maintain healthy beautiful nails. As we know that olive oil is rich in polyphenols with anti bacterial and anti fungal properties olive oil is good to moisturize and strengthen the fragile fingernails.

Methods of using Olive Oil:

Treats Brittle Nails: Nails become brittle when they dry up. As the nails lack oil and sweat glands, it is very important to moisturize the nails. Massage with olive oil every night to treat brittle nails naturally. Do this thrice a week to treat brittle nails.

Soft Nails: To get soft nails, mix olive oil with honey. Mix and apply on the nails as well as cuticles. Leave for 10 minutes and then rinse with cold water. Pat dry with a towel. Do this twice every week to care for nails and make them soft.

Nail Growth: This is another use of olive oil for nail care. Mix olive oil with tomato pulp or juice. Apply on the nails as well as cuticles. You can also soak your nails in the mix for 10-15 minutes. Rinse with cold water and pat dry. Do this twice a week to increase nail growth easily. Tomato contains biotin which increases growth of nails naturally.

Soft Cuticles: Dry and rough cuticles are a turn off! For proper nail care, use olive oil. Apply it on the cuticles and nails after bath and before going to bed. Do this every day to care for your nails.

Dry Nails: To treat dry nails, apply olive oil three times a day. It will not just treat dry nails, but also make them shiny. If applied on palms too, olive oil will soften the skin.

Strengthen Nails With Olive Oil:

- Soak your fingernails in olive oil once or twice a week. Warm half a cup of extra virgin olive oil in a bowl and plunge your fingernails for a 10-15 minute soak. Olive oil will be absorbed into the fingernails, cuticle and surrounding skin which will impart the moisture and strength to your damaged, brittle and peeling nails.

- You can massage your nails and fingers with warm olive oil on daily basis. It helps to retain the moisture besides boosting the blood circulation and giving your nails a natural shine.

- Olive oil is also good for your cuticles and so used in many nail salons. After using a nail polish remover, it is a good idea to rub some olive oil over your nails and fingers. It will help to keep the nails and cuticles soft and intact.

- This great oil also works great for your nail growth. Mix half a cup of tomato juice with 2 tablespoons of olive oil in a shallow bowl and soak your fingers for 10 minutes, before rinsing your hands off. While tomato juice help the growth of nails, olive oil imparts the moisture to nails and cuticles.

- Extra virgin olive oil massage is ideal for dry nails and cuticles. Forego the expensive hand and cuticle creams, instead massage a couple of olive oil drops onto the cuticles and around the nails. Its regular use will make your cuticles stay moist and nails shiny.

- Alternatively, give a warm olive oil bath to your nails. It's a great way to strengthen them. It will take just 5-10 minutes. Simply soak your nails in a slightly warm olive oil. Remember not to heat it too much, as it loses its properties at high temperature. Apply this olive oil nails treatment once or twice a week to strengthen your nails. With this treatment they will also look healthy and shiny.

- When you apply olive oil on your nail beds, it acts as a moisturizer. It keeps them soft and healthy so they don't start to peel off and make your nails look dry and un-kept. And it's always a plus when you can stay away from whitlow.

- Applying olive oil to your nails gives it great shine just like it does your hair. All you have to do is soak them in olive oil for 20-30 minutes and then buff with a flat cotton pad. After this you can place them in a soft fiber glove or keep them still for a few minutes before you carry on with your other activities.

Other Uses of Olive Oil

1. Shaving Cream Alternative:

For both men and women, olive oil can be applied to the area to be shaved. Thanks to the oiliness of the olive oil, it can help to avoid razor bumps and even cuts from the razor. Rub olive oil onto the face or body, until glistening and then shave as normal.

2. Relief from Eczema:

Thanks to the moisturizing properties of olive oil, using this for eczema is great. Simply rub some olive oil into the palms of hands and rub on the affected areas.

3. Stop the Squeaky Door:

If you have a squeaky door, simply place a few drops of olive oil on the hinges, and the squeak will be gone.

4. Remove Makeup from Eyes:

Simply put olive oil onto a cotton ball and swipe across the eye lid to remove any eye makeup that is being used. It is a safe, gentle and effective solution to use.

5. A Great Polish:

Inexpensive when compared to furniture polish, olive oil can help to add the gleam and shine back into furniture. Simply put this on a cloth and wipe over the furniture to be polished. It can also be used on silver and gold to bring out the shine.

6. Help Ear Wax:

If you suffer with ear wax buildup, place a few drops of olive oil into the ears at night for a few nights. In 3 to 4 nights, the ear wax will break up and be easier to remove.

7. Treat Diaper Rash:

Babies have delicate skin, but olive oil can be used as a great diaper rash treatment. Simply rub this onto the affected area, and overnight the rash will start to heal.

8. Clean Makeup Brushes:

In order to be effective, makeup brushes have to be cleaned from time to time. Olive oil combined with antibacterial soap can remove any and all makeup that may be caked into the brush.

9. Nonstick Zippers:

When jackets get older or due to wear and tear, zippers can become stuck from time to time. Use a cotton tip with olive oil to rub on the zipper. The zipper will start to move with ease afterwards.

10. Fix Heels of Feet:

Cracked heels are often embarrassing and uncomfortable. After using a pumice stone on the heels, soak olive oil on your heels, then wear socks all night to lock in the moisture.

ACKNOWLEDGMENT

We live in a world of beauty, charm and adventure.

There shouldn't be an end to our adventures. And the

easiest adventure is to save or regain our beauty by

getting inspired by this beautiful world we are living in.

'Olive Oil'

is meant to be one of those beauties of nature.

Legend has it that the olive tree was a gift from the GOD.

Homer referred to olive oil as liquid gold, and Thomas

Jefferson proclaimed it the richest gift of heaven. For

centuries, a gift of olive oil was a welcome treasure.

Food-lovers have never entirely forgotten the delightful

golden fluid, but in recent years, a new awareness of the

benefits of olive oil has been born. Science has turned its

investigative eye upon it in recent years, and numerous

studies have only reinforced the notion that olive oil is an amazing substance with numerous benefits. The above are some of those olive oil benefits I came up with my personal experience.

If you loved this book and found it useful I would be very glad if you post a short review. I read all the reviews personally so I can get your feedback and make this book even better.

THANK YOU

AVA COLLINS

www.ingramcontent.com/pod-product-compliance
Lightning Source LLC
Chambersburg PA
CBHW050758290526
45792CB00008B/2235